Table of Content

Copyright

Fra Fra's Naturals
13 N. Washington St
Ste. 189
Ypsilanti, MI 48197
Info@frafrasnaturals.com
www.frafrasnaturals.com

Printed in the United States of America
First printing, 2020

This eBook contains information that has been carefully researched and examined for accuracy. It is intended to help the readers be better informed consumers of skin care products. It is presented as general advice. This book is not intended to be a substitute for the medical advice of a licensed dermatologist. The reader should consult with their doctor in any matters relating to his/her health. The information provided within this eBook is for general informational purposes only. While we try to keep the information up-to-date and correct, there are no representations or warranties, express or implied, about the completeness, accuracy, reliability, suitability or availability with respect to the information, products, services, or related graphics contained in this eBook for any purpose. Any use of this information is at your own risk.

INTRODUCTION

At Fra Fra's Naturals we believe that natural is better. We not only sell African black soap and shea butter, but we are faithful users as well. My husband and I began this journey several years ago to alleviate our daughter's eczema symptoms and help my elderly mother-in-law who needed something to protect her fragile skin.

My daughter used to scratch grooves in her skin when her eczema flared up. It was hard to see her in so much discomfort and nothing the doctor prescribed was effective. I vividly remember taking her to the pediatrician and they prescribed her Eucerin mixed with hydrocortisone cream. I was shocked when her doctor gave me the warnings:

    1. May thin skin and cause skin sensitivity

    2. Can bleach skin

    3. Can cause blistering

    4. Can cause increased redness, swelling and itchiness

I immediately wondered - what am I exposing my daughter to? Before this point I'd never considered how safe our skin care was. It had never even entered my mind to wonder about skin care ingredients and side effects.

When I shared my concerns with my husband, he began searching for something that could help our daughter and his mother without the negative side effects and thus obsession with African black soap and shea butter began. As we learned more about African black soap and Shea Butter and saw the difference it made in our hair and skin firsthand, we wanted to share our experiences with our friends and family, but no one really knew what African black soap and Shea Butter was. We got a lot of push back at first:

- Is Shea Butter good for your face?

- It's too thick it will give me acne!
- It's too greasy! I'm going to be shiny all day!
- That stuff doesn't work! It's all a gimmick!

But once people tried it, they loved it! The only complaint was that it was hard to apply in it's raw form. Always up to a challenge we devised a patent pending process that allowed us to whip shea butter to a light, airy consistency without heating it or refining it, allowing the shea butter to retain all of its benefits. Our whipped Shea Butter was a hit! We knew then that there was a lot of misconception about African black soap and whipped Shea butter that needed to be clarified. The purpose of this book is to educate you, the reader, about authentic, raw, unrefined African Shea butter.

As a bonus we have included 10 super easy diy skin care recipes that utilizes Shea butter as its base. I strongly believe in all-natural skin care but sometimes it can be a little pricey so we have developed some recipes we could do at home and now we are sharing these recipes with you so let's get started!

CHAPTER ONE:

WHAT IS SHEA BUTTER?

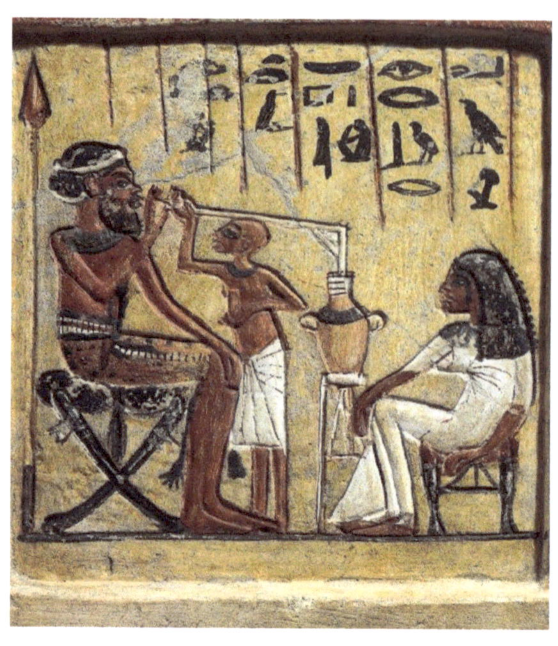

Africa has a wealth of natural resources and generational wisdom. Ancient Africans in what is now known as Egypt, South Africa, and Nigeria were far more advanced scientifically than any other civilization Unfortunately, the history of great scientific accomplishments of ancient Africans has largely gone unrecognized. Ancient African medical literature is among the oldest in existence and in 2014 researchers described the ancient Africans understanding of the cardiovascular system as "surprisingly sophisticated." History shows that many scientific achievements of Ancient Africans comprised of the use of plants for restorative purposes. In fact, the knowledge and uses of essential oils were introduced to the world by the ancient Egyptians Additionally, medical procedures such as abortions, autopsies, brain surgery, bone setting, and cataract surgery were being done in ancient Africa long before they were being performed by western practitioners.

This extensive knowledge of the use of plants is what lead to the creation of the powerhouse Shea butter.

Shea butter is an all-natural, plant-based moisturizer that has numerous health benefits. This butter is known to help people manage problem skin such as: Acne, Psoriasis, dermatitis, dark spots and eczema. It is naturally infused with high concentrations of vitamins A and E. Currently it is handmade by the local women in Western Africa with the bulk being produced in Ghana.

The type of oils used, and the exact method of production depends upon the region in which it is made.

Did you know that Shea butter was Cleopatra's go to beauty product? Yes, there are historical records that shows that Cleopatra was obsessed with Shea butter. In fact, anytime she traveled she would take caravans of jars filled with Shea butter and Shea nuts with her. She used it for her skin and hair.

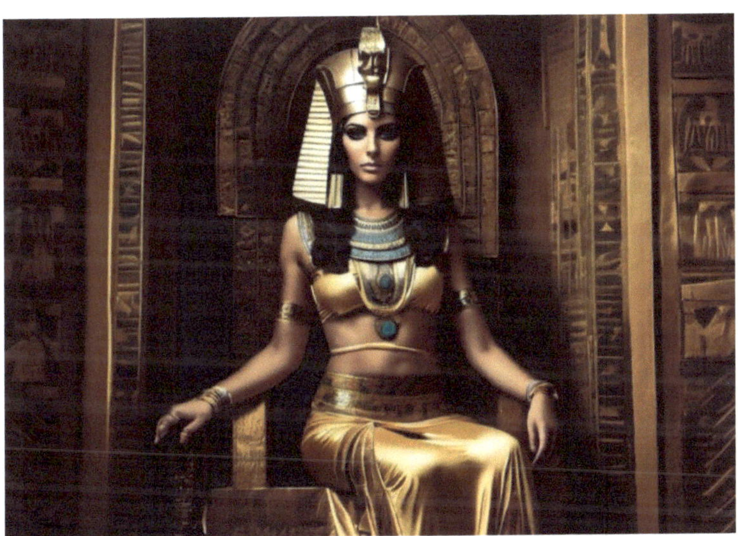

Cleopatra was smarter than she was beautiful. She was a published author and wrote a medical treatise called "cosmetic" which included recipes for skincare products to help with skin conditions. Of course, this is the woman that successfully seduced two of the most powerful men in the world so one must assume she knew a little something about beauty and skincare but Shea butter goes way back before even Cleopatra. Ancient Africans used Shea butter to protect their skin and hair from the harsh sun and sooth insect bites.

The Shea tree (Vitellaria paradoxa) is native to western and central Africa. The tree is known as "the tree of life" because every part of the tree has either a health or community benefit. The sap from the tree is a very efficient glue, the bark is used as a remedy for tummy aches, the branches are chewed on to clean teeth and treat gum disease (surprising fact: the benefits derived from chewing on the branch of a Shea tree is equal to or greater than the benefits derived from toothpaste). The fruit of the tree, the shea fruit, has a texture like berries and is delicious and nutritious and used in numerous traditional recipes.

This amazing tree is also called "Women's Gold" because the production of Shea butter is traditionally women's work. In some parts of African men are not allowed to even touch the Shea tree at all. Only women can harvest the fruit and gather materials. Once the Shea fruit has been eaten the nuts are collected to produce Shea butter. The recipe for authentic Shea butter is a tightly guarded secret. The only way to know the recipe is if it has been passed down through the generations but the exact recipe is unknown outside of the villages.

So how is Shea butter such a beauty staple if the original recipe can't be reproduced? Well, like anything else valuable there are knock offs. Yes, yes, there are fake Shea butters and there are subpar Shea butters. The shea butter base used by commercial skin care companies are refined beyond hope and fractionated. This means that the Shea butter has been exposed to high heat, the color and the natural nutty smokey smell has been removed and then it has been liquified. What remains is a small portion of Shea butters natural healing properties.

CHAPTER TWO:

HOW IS SHEA BUTTER MADE?

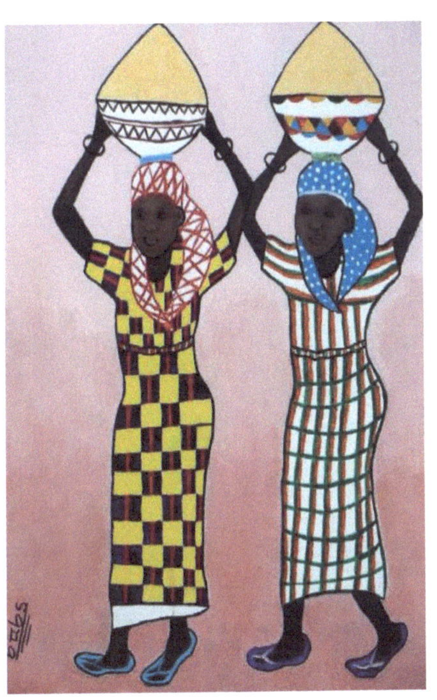

The main ingredient in Shea butter is the butter from the seed/nut of the Shea fruit. The nuts are collected and sorted to remove undesirable nuts, washed and parboiled for 30 minutes and then laid out to dry in the sun for hours. Once the nuts are dry, they are removed from the shell and dried for a second time and then sorted again for a third time getting rid of any inferior nuts.

Now the nuts are crushed and roasted for 30 minutes until enough water has been removed from the nuts to allow them to be crushed into a fine powder. Water is then added, and the paste is kneaded into a creamy paste. It is beaten and stirred by hand for hours while water is slowly added.

Eventually a layer of fatty oil separates from the paste and rises to the top in curd-like clumps. The clumps of oil are removed and is washed up to 5 times to sanitize it before it is boiled once again to remove excess moisture. Pure liquified Shea butter rises to the top and is gathered, filtered and poured into another bowl and allowed to cool. The resulting Shea butter will be off- white or cream in color however, depending on the extraction method, it can range from off white to yellow or even light green.

HEALING FRACTIONS OF OILS COMMONLY USED IN SKINCARE PRODUCTS

BABY OIL	0%
MINERAL OIL	0%
CASTOR OIL	0.2 – 0.3%
AVOCADO OIL	0.5 – 2.5%
OLIVE OIL	1.0 – 2.0%
ARGAN OIL	1.5 – 3.5%
REFINED SHEA BUTTER	1.0 – 3.0%
AVOCADO OIL	2.0 – 6.0%
COCOA BUTTER	3.0
GRADE B SHEA BUTTER	4.0 - 9.0%
JOJOBA OIL	4.0 – 9.0%
COCONUT OIL	15%
COCOA BUTTER	5.0 -15.0%
SUNFLOWER OIL	15%
GRADE A SHEA BUTTER	17%

CHAPTER THREE:

SO, WHAT IS SO SPECIAL ABOUT SHEA BUTTER?

If you look around at body butters, lotions and creams you will notice that the ones that include Shea butter are considered high end and generally cost more. This is because it is widely known that Shea butter is undeniably different from any other natural ingredient. Scientist have analyzed this and what it comes down to is raw Shea butters Healing Fraction or unsaponifiable fraction. Shea butter has a larger healing fraction than most natural ingredients used in skin care products. Shea butters healing fraction rate ranges from 5% to 17% while other oils, nuts and seeds come in at about 1%. With healing power like this it is no wonder that Shea butter is so revered. It provides more overall health benefits than any other product out there.

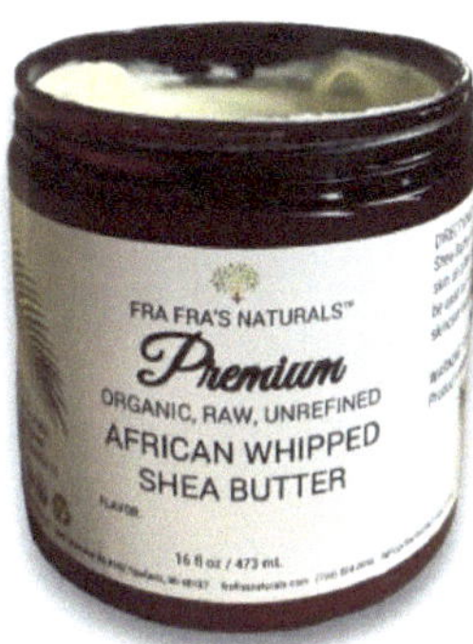

Raw Shea Butter is rich in Oleic Acid, Stearic Acid, Palmitic Acid, Linoleic Acid, Cinnamic Acid Esters, Allantoin, and Polyphenols, and vitamins A,B,C,D,E,F and K. To break it down further let's look at ratio of fatty acids found in Shea Butter:

- 45-50% **Oleic Acid** - Exceptional for dry and aging skin because it easily penetrates deep into the skin's layers replacing the skins moisture. It can also restore the natural oil of skin, without clogging pores.

- 30-40% **Stearic Acid** – a fatty acid that has been shown to act as a protective moisture barrier.

- 5-9% **Palmitic Acid** - it locks moisture into your skin rather than letting it evaporate. As we age our skin looses up to 31% of its naturals reserves of this acid.

- 4-5% **Linoleic Acid (Vitamin F)** - Linoleic acid is an essential fatty acid that your body can't produce. This fatty acid is normally reserved for premium skin care products because it is known to reverse UV radiation damage, increase moisture and barrier function, even out skin tone, increase circulation and cellular production.

- 1.3- 7.5% **Cinnamic Acid Esters** – This fatty acid is an antioxidant and is also antimicrobial. It has skin lightening properties and is beneficial to aging skin because it stimulates collagen production.

Allantoin is responsible for Shea Butters natural anti-inflammatory property. It soothes and calms irritated skin and has been used to help heal wounds because it increases the cellular regeneration rate.

The **Polyphenols** content is responsible for Shea Butters ability to protect the skin from oxidative stress thus preventing signs of aging and may possibly aid in inhibiting skin cancer.

The **Vitamin A** found in Shea Butter is naturally occurring and in complete synergy with the rest of the fatty acids. This is essential because Vitamin A necessary to maintain healthy, balanced and even-toned skin. It encourages healthy skin cell turnover which prevents dead skin cells from clogging pores. It is also good for skin conditions such as eczema and psoriasis, which is characterized by rough, scaly, dry skin because it is believed to be potential signs of a vitamin A deficiency in the skin.

The **Vitamin C** (ascorbic acid) plays an important role in creation of collagen and skin health. even out skin tone and diminish the appearance of fine lines and wrinkles. This powerful vitamin is known as a skin brightener but even more impressive is its ability to shield skin from environmental toxins and free radical damage.

Vitamin D plays an important role in supporting the skin barrier as well as the skin's immune system and wound healing. A vitamin D deficiency can cause some significant side effects. It can lead to serious skin conditions including but not limited to: psoriasis and atopic dermatitis. Vitamin D is also essential to maintain healthy hair and the hair growth cycle. There is a link between having a vitamin D deficiency and developing alopecia.

Ah, **Vitamin E/Tocopherol**…My mom used Vitamin E pills to get me through middle school. I swear my acne making hormones must have been in overdrive. If the number of pimples you can fit on a forehead was an Olympic sport, I would be a gold medalist many times over. Vitamin E is a restorative. It strengthens the skins moisture barrier function, natural anti-inflammatory, a moderately effective UV screen, reduces scarring and dark spots. Additionally, vitamin E is an antioxidant which means it seeks out and kills free radicals.

Vitamin K is an overlooked but plays a vital role in maintaining healthy glowing skin. You see vitamin K is a healing agent. It helps to heal bruises quickly, increases recovery time after trauma or a procedure. It also helps reduce inflammation, redness, puffy eyes and under eye circles.

Even better, it makes your skin more resilient! It is what gives Shea butter its ability to minimize scars, fade stretch marks and reduce the appearance of spider veins.

CHAPTER FOUR:

10 POWERFUL BENEFITS OF SHEA BUTTER

It is pretty obvious from the previous chapter why Shea Butter is such a sought-after skin care ingredient, but does it live up to its reputation? Let me answer that question for you – Yes, Yes, a Thousand Times, Yes! Whatever you heard about Shea Butter that led you to read this book is true and probably more. We have already discussed its moisturizing, anti-aging, antimicrobial, antibacterial, anti-inflammatory and healing properties but there is still sooooo much more to this miracle butter.

- *Antifungal* - Shea tree products have been clinically proven to fight fungal infections. While it does not kill all fungi, it is effective when treating the common fungi that causes ringworm and athletes feet.

- *Balances sebum levels* – Not only does shea butter restore moisture deep down into the lower levels of the skin it also helps skin maintain its natural sebum levels, discouraging over production consequently reducing acne breakouts.

- *Prevents hair breakage* – It is important to note that Shea butter is an emollient that has moisturizing properties. Many people apply Shea butter to the ends of their hair before shampooing. This keeps the ends soft to prevent breakage and splitting.

- *Protects damaged hair* - If you have hair that is damaged from heat or styling simply you can use Shea butter as a hair mask. Apply Shea butter to hair and wrap your head in a warm damp towel. Leave it in for 30 minutes and then wash and condition as usual.

- *Rids scalp of dandruff* – If you have a bad case of the dandruff flakes you can apply Shea butter directly to the scalp. Applying Shea butter directly to the scalp decreases dandruff and moisturizes hair follicles.

- *Soothes arthritis* – Arthritis is inflammation of the sacs between the joints. Shea butter is such a powerful anti-inflammatory that a 2016 study on knee joints showed that applying shea butter to the knee considerably lowered inflammation and protected the knee joints from further damage.

- *Relieves nasal congestion* – Uh huh, you read that right. Shea butter is a clinically proven nasal decongestant. A study conducted in 1979 showed that when applied to the inside nostrils and around the bridge it is more effective at clearing airways than traditional nasal drops.

- *Lowers cholesterol* – Shea butter is a natural vegetable oil and is excellent for cooking. A study done by the American Journal of Clinical Nutrition shows that the high stearic acid content found in Shea butter, when ingested, reduces lipoprotein and plasma cholesterol levels. Shea butter is routinely used in recipes in African countries.

- *Treats diarrhea* – Got bathroom issues? Eating Shea

butter is a traditional African remedy to treat diarrhea, dysentery and other gastrointestinal issues.

- *Alleviates Razor Bumps* – Shea butter is often used by men to alleviate razor bumps and ingrown hair that can occur after shaving. When shea butter is used prior to shaving it protects and softens the skin reducing the likelihood of razor bumps.

CHAPTER FIVE:

HOW TO USE RAW SHEA BUTTER

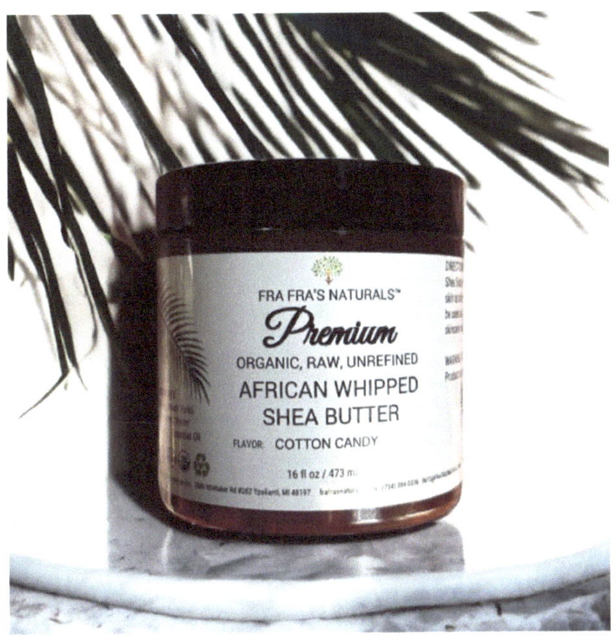

Shea Butter has a well-deserved reputation as a miracle butter. It has many versatile uses and can be used to treat ailments both externally and internally. How many other butters can you say that about? When I was first introduced to Shea butter, I just slathered it all over my daughter.

She looked like she had been dipped in a giant bucket of fried chicken. Personally, I was using it for EVERYTHING including hair grease. I learned after my hair turned to straw that there is a right way and a wrong way to use Shea Butter.

Do a skin test first!

Always do a skin test when switching to a new skin care product. It is possible to have a reaction to Shea Butter if you are allergic to tree nuts. No tree but reactions have ever been reported but it still important to consider this. To do a skin test apply a small amount to your inner wrist. If a rash or swelling occurs or you develop breathing problems seek emergency treatment immediately.

How to use Shea Butter on your face

Shea butter in its raw form can be applied directly to your face but can be difficult to spread. A light, airy Shea butter whipped with organic oils (like Fra Fra's Naturals organic raw whipped Shea butter) is a great product to add to your skin care routine. Here is a good nighttime routine:

STEP ONE – Wash your face

Wash your face with a gently cleanser such as liquid African Black soap to free your skin from the dirt, impurities and environmental toxins that accumulated on your skin during the day. Using a good cleanser will allow you to get a deep clean to unclog pores without stripping the skin of its natural oils. Do not skimp on your cleanser to save a few extra bucks. It's really not worth it and your skin will pay for it in the end. Make sure to read the labels and understand which each ingredient is and what it does. If you can't pronounce it, you don't need it.

STEP TWO – Apply a toner

A toner is a liquid solution designed to follow your cleanser to make sure that any pollutants still lingering after your face washing. It is also used to rid your skin of dead cells on your skin's surface that leads to acne and black heads while restoring your its pH balance. Look for a toner that has wholesome ingredients like aloe vera, rose water, vitamin E or even chamomile tea. If you're dealing with aging skin perhaps you want a toner that includes hyaluronic acid. To use apply soak a cotton ball with toner and wipe your entire face and neck and chest with it.

STEP THREE – Serum

This is strictly a nighttime step because many serums don't do good when exposed to sunlight. They can either become ineffective or they can become a skin irritant. Neither option is particularly appealing so nighttime only it is. Now this is not a necessary step. It is completely optional, but it is a good way to address acne, fine lines and wrinkles and dark spots. Serums with retinal, fruit stem cells, peptides, or Alpha Hydroxy Acids are all good antiaging options. Serums with Vitamins A and E are particularly good for brightening dull skin. If you are fighting acne try a serum that has ingredients such as salicylic acid, Alpha Hydroxy Acids or Beta Hydroxy Acid. You could even go for a serum that has botanical extracts like grapefruit extract, broccoli extract, cucumber or the all mighty Tea Tree oil.

STEP FOUR – Moisturize

The last step in your nighttime routine should be a good moisturizer. This is where Shea butter shines. Shea butter will seal in all of the hydrating and moisturizing ingredients that has already been applied to your face and neck. Shea butter is the best choice because it is full of natural vitamins and fatty acids that further increase moisture levels and you will wake up with the coveted glow the next morning.

How to use Shea Butter for your lips

Your lips need just as much care and attention as your skin. Shea butter can be used as a lip balm on dry chapped lips. It absorbs easily and offers vital nutrients and moisture that lips need especially during the dry winter months. When the wind is howling, and temperatures dip Shea butter will seal in moisture and create a barrier to keep your lips supple.

How to use Shea Butter to minimize razor burn and hair bumps

Both men and women shave to get rid of unwanted hair. A razor is the most common tool used to achieve this goal, but it comes with its short comings. The use of a razor often leads to itchy, irritated, bumpy skin. Applying Shea butter the day before shaving will soften your skin which can assist in reducing the chance of developing razor bumps and ingrown hairs. It will also make skin smoother so that shaving is easier and does not leave skin raw and irritated.

How to use Shea Butter to heal wounds

As you've already read, the vitamin K content found in Shea Butter is excellent at healing wounds. You can apply Shea Butter to cuts, burns, and incisions to decrease healing time and avoid an unsightly scar. This is not to mean you won't have any scarring. Often that is unavoidable. Only that Shea butter will lessen the appearance of said scar. Shea Butter will skin deep into the subdermal layers of skin and deliver vital fatty acids that will repair cells and boost the production of new skin cells. .

How to use Shea Butter to control frizzy hair

Shea butter can be used as a hair styling product if you have dry, coarse and/or frizzy hair. Merely take a bit of Shea butter and smooth it through your hair to tame flyways. It will give your hair a nice healthy shine and reduce the frizzing to a manageable amount.

CHAPTER SIX:

RAW SHEA BUTTER FOR OILY SKIN

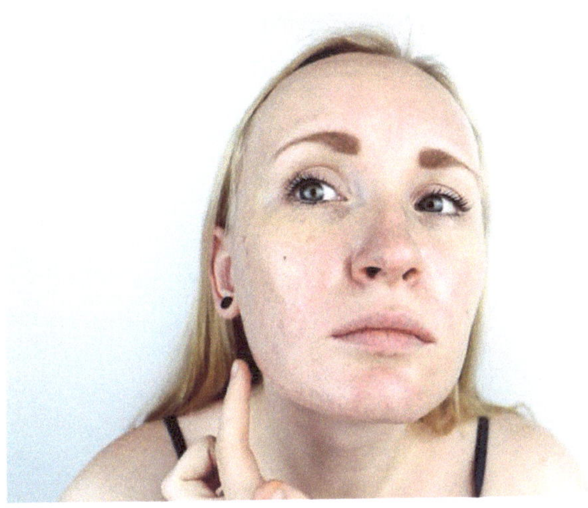

Oily skin is the direct result of the overproduction of sebum from sebaceous glands located under the skin's surface. When these glands are overactive it can lead to oily skin causing thicker skin that tends to look greasy. It can also lead to clogged pores and a tendency to break out with acne. Hormonal changes, genetics, diet, stress or even certain medications can increase sebum production. However, there are some positive aspects of having oily skin. Oily skin does not age at the same rate as other skin types. Oily skin is also less prone to premature aging so yay for that!

Some people avoid oil-based moisturizers for fear of breaking out. The belief is that adding oil to oily skin is bad. This is a misnomer. If you take the time to find the correct plant-based oil based moisturizer it will help to control or even lessen the sebum your skin produces. It might seem counterintuitive but it's true. Adding the right oil to oily skin will make it less oily. Now take a minute and let that sink in Okay, so now you should be wondering "is Shea butter the correct oil?" and the answer is YES!

Shea Butter has a comedogenic rating of 0. Comedogenic means any product that blocks or clogs pores and causes black heads and or breakouts. The comedogenic scale rates products from 0 to 5.Shea butter is one of a very select few plants based moisturizes that has no comedogenic effect. Instead of clogging pores Shea butter sinks deep into the lower layers of skin and plumps and hydrates while balancing out your sebum production therefore correcting the problem. As a bonus raw Shea butter has antiaging properties.

CHAPTER SEVEN:

RAW SHEA BUTTER FOR SENSITIVE/REACTIVE SKIN

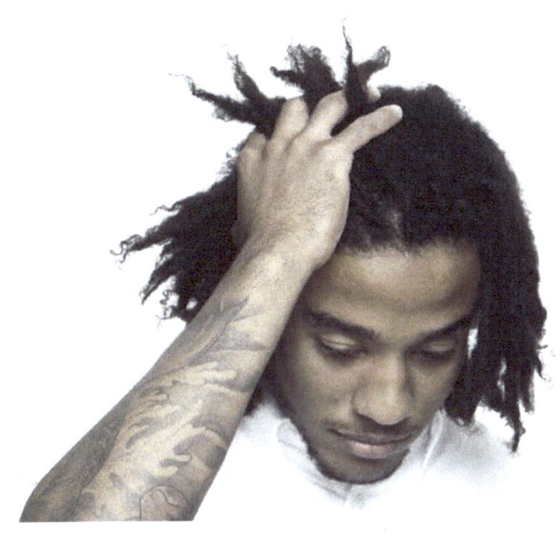

Sensitive skin is thin and may have dry patches. This skin type is sensitive to temperature changes, becomes easily irritated, burns easily and has a prone to allergic reaction. Some studies suggest that sensitive reactive skin is due to all the pollutants, and toxic irritants found in modern cosmetics and skin care. If you have sensitive reactive skin you should avoid using products that have dyes, perfumes, preservatives or chemicals.

Raw Shea butter is made with plant-based ingredients and is completely devoid of pollutants and toxins. Even though it is a nut product it typically does not trigger nut allergies. There has not been a documented case of an allergic attack due to Shea butter. That is not to mean that there will never be one. If you have a nut allergy you should be cautious and hyper aware of any changes after doing a skin patch test. If you can tolerate Shea butter you will find that it is one of the most soothing products you will find for sensitive skin. It is calming, hydrating and nourishing. It will maintain your skins pH balance and strengthen your skins moisture barrier thus protecting it from those dreaded environmental toxins I referenced earlier.

CHAPTER EIGHT:
RAW SHEA BUTTER FOR DRY SKIN

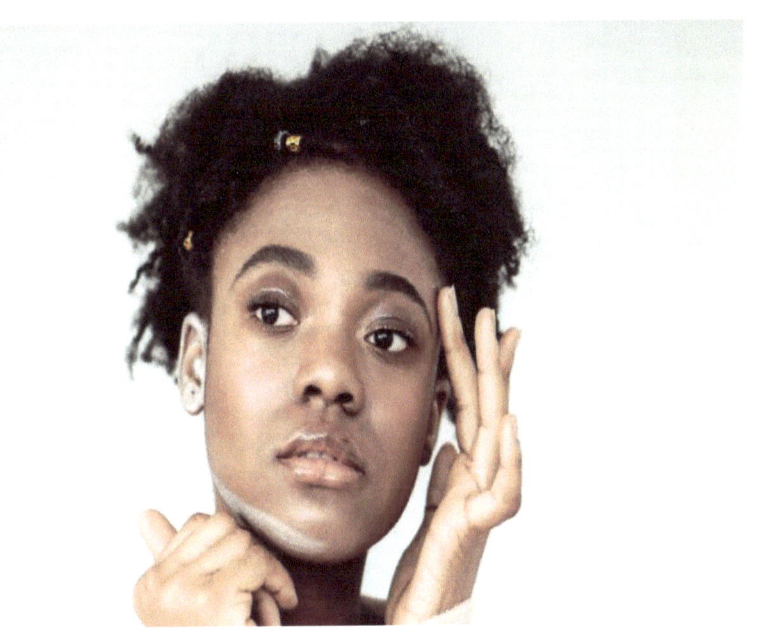

Dry skin can be a pain. This skin type can have dry itchy flaky patches, feel uncomfortable after cleansing and can age prematurely. On the flip side dry skin has smaller pores that are virtually invisible. Dry skin sufferers tend to spend a lot of money on moisturizers and skin care trying to get smoother, softer skin. Naturally Shea butter can help with that.

The stearic, palmitic, and linoleic acids help strengthen the skin barrier and locks in the much- needed moisture that dry skin lacks. It is not sticky and absorbs quickly which means you can reapply it several times throughout the day without repercussions. It is easy to use and is a good base to use if you are into creating your own beauty products to avoid triggering your skin.

CHAPTER NINE:

RAW SHEA BUTTER FOR SKIN CONDITIONS

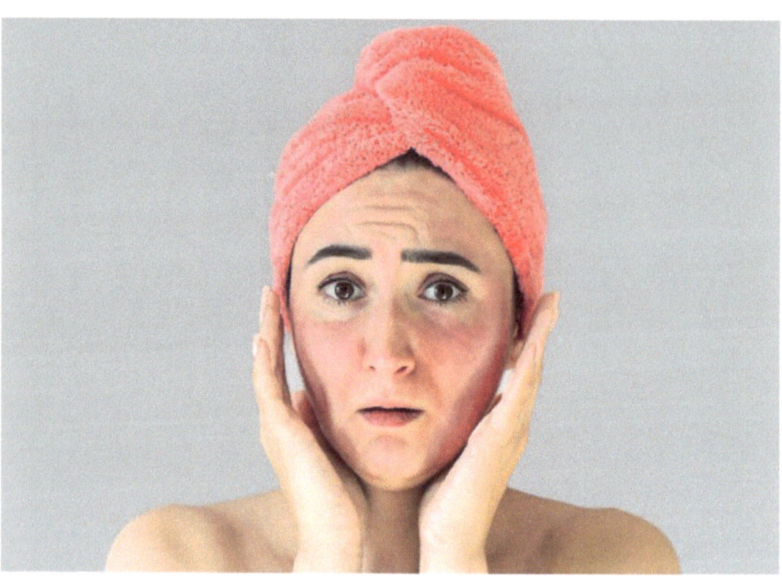

Raw Shea Butter is often used to treat a variety of skin conditions. It is effective for treating rosacea, eczema, dermatitis, psoriasis, rashes, fungal infections, burns and other inflammatory conditions. It is gentle, anti-inflammatory, antibacterial and has healing properties as well. The ample amount of vitamin E is a major reason why it works.

Vitamin E is added to many skin care products. Unfortunately, the benefits of the added vitamin E in over-the-counter moisturizers are often diminished by chemical additives. Raw Shea Butter does not have any chemical additives or preservatives thus retaining the vitamin E and its benefits. It is good for problem skin that is dry and patchy and reduces or stops itchiness. Shea Butter provides deep down and lasting hydration to the skin. It moisturizes and conditions the skin slowing, and sometimes even stopping, the reoccurrence of eczema, rosacea, and psoriasis. Moreover, Shea Butter fights inflammation and soothes the swelling and pain that often accompanies a flare-up.

CHAPTER TEN:

WHY AND HOW TO BUY RAW UNREFINED SHEA BUTTER

Buying authentic raw unrefined Shea Butter can be confusing. Skin care manufacturers know about the healing properties of Shea Butter and like with any popular product there are a lot of imitations on the market. This is to be expect as the old saying goes "Imitation is the greatest form of flattery." And while that may be true it is definitely not good for the consumer. Fake or refined Shea butter does not have the same healing properties as the raw unrefined Shea Butter does. If you are searching for Shea butter, you want to make sure that you're getting what you're paying for. You will find Shea Butter listed as an ingredient in many shampoos and moisturizers. What the ingredient list does not tell you is the grade of Shea Butter that is used and whether it is processed or not.

Why should I care if it is raw and unrefined or not?

Real Shea Butter cannot be made outside of Africa. This is because it is an ancient recipe that is religiously guarded and has not been shared outside of the village women. This shouldn't be a problem, but Shea Butter has a natural nutty, smoky smell and the color ranges from ivory to yellow. (Quick side note: There are imitation yellow Shea butters on the market. I will discuss those later). To make it more appealing to consumers manufactures seek to remove the color and smell of raw Shea Butter. They do this by creating refined Shea Butter in large manufacturing plants. The process they use to create this butter is destructive. They use a substance called hexane or they may use petroleum solvents. The butter is then boiled, heated to more than 400 degrees Fahrenheit to remove the toxic solvents that they themselves introduced to the butter. But wait there is more…It is bleached, BLEACHED, and exposed to Sodium Hydroxide to remove the color and smell of the Shea butter. By the time the process is complete you can't even consider the finished product as real Shea Butter. The boiling and bleaching process effectively removed all of the benefits associated with unrefined Shea butter.

What are the pros and cons of using raw unrefined Shea Butter vs Refined Shea Butter?

Pros of using raw Shea Butter	Cons of using raw Shea Butter
<ul><li>Has the maximum amount of bioactive phytochemicals present</li><li>Antioxidants that are beneficial for skin are protected</li><li>The benefits from the Vitamin E (what makes it off-white or yellow) present</li><li>Soft and malleable</li><li>Does not contain preservatives or fragrances.</li><li>Absorbs completely within minutes and does not leave a greasy residue</li></ul>	<ul><li>Odorless and colorless</li><li>Easier to apply</li><li>Easy to use as a base for lotions and creams</li><li>Less expensive</li></ul>

Cons of using raw Shea Butter	Cons of using raw Shea Butter
• May contain flecks of impurities (unprocessed ingredients) • Difficult to use as a base for lotions and creams due to its thick consistency. • Has a distinctive smoky nutty smell. • Can be hard to apply in its raw form.	• Hard and grainy • Most bioactive phytochemicals and antioxidants have been lost during manufacturing • Increased chance of allergic reaction and/or skin irritation as a result of exposure to chemicals and fragrances.

How can I tell if it is raw or refined?

- Raw Shea Butter should be Free Trade and certified organic.

- Refined Shea Butter will have additives and/or fragrances in the ingredient list.

- Raw Shea Butter is unshaped and even in a container (unless it is whipped) it will have a uniform shape.

- Raw Shea Butter will melt upon touch.

- Refined Shea Butter will be hard and grainy.

- The best and most important way to make sure you are purchasing raw Shea butter is to purchase it from a trusted vendor.

Decoding Shea butter Grades

GRADE A	Raw or unrefined. Extracted using water. Ivory or beige in color. Contains the highest ratio of Shea nuts and bioactive nutrients. Can be consumed and used in cosmetics. Shelf stable for more than a year. This is the only grade of Shea butter with a healing fraction of 17%.
GRADE B	Can be refined or unrefined. Color ranges from ivory to yellow. Has a smaller ratio of Shea nuts and bioactive nutrients than Grade A. Cannot be consumed but it is good for cosmetics. Shelf stable for more than a year.
GRADE C	Highly refined. Extracted with chemical solvents like Hexane. White in color. Contains a low level of Shea nuts and bioactive nutrients. Cannot be consumed. Most widely used in commercial cosmetics. Shelf stable for more than a year.
GRADE D	Can be refined or unrefined. Color ranges from ivory to yellow. Lowest uncontaminated grade with the lowest level of bioactive nutrients. It is not shelf stable and will go rancid within a few months.
GRADE E	Raw or unrefined but contains undesirable

contaminants such as feces, mold, parasites or mildew. Not safe for consumer use or consumption.

Ivory vs Yellow Shea Butter

As discussed, Shea butter varies in color from ivory to light yellow. The different colors denote where the butter was made and slight variations in the recipe. If bark of the borututu tree is added during the Shea butter making process it will dye the shea butter yellow. The borututu bark has similar properties to the shea nut in it is full of antioxidants and helps with skin problems like eczema and dermatitis. Both Ivory and yellow Shea butter can be authentic, and either is good for all skin types.

Fake Yellow Shea Butter

There are yellow butters on the market that are labeled as Shea butter but in reality, it is Kpangnan butter or African butter. This butter is made from the Butter tree (Pentadesma butyracea). This tree grows in the rainforest and on the riverbanks in West Africa. It has been traded internationally for years as yellow or golden Shea butter. In truth these butters have marked differences. Their fatty acid profiles are comparable, but their bioactive fractions differ. Shea butters bioactive fraction is between 300 – 400 times larger than that of African Butter.

How can I tell if it is Shea butter or African butter?

African butter is a mustard yellow and closely resembles Shea butter. Here are some easy ways to know what you are buying:

- African butter is hard like cocoa butter and doesn't melt easily like Shea butter.

- It has a firm powdery texture when stored at room temperature

- African butter smells like a mix between cocoa butter and shea butter

CHAPTER ELEVEN:

SHEA BUTTER FAQ'S

How Do I Store Shea Butter?

Shea butter should be stored in a dry cool place away from heat and direct sunlight. If you have a large amount of Shea butter you can store it in the refrigerator to extend the shelf life. Keep in mind that refrigerating Shea butter will make it hard.

My Shea Butter Melted

Shea butter is vulnerable to fluctuating temperatures. If Shea butter is stored in a car or transported during the summer months, it will liquify. The good thing is that the healing properties of the melted Shea butter is intact. Shea butter is so soft that it melts at right about the normal body temperature. If your Shea Butter melts you can either put it in the refrigerator or store it in a dark cool place and allow it to solidify. Be sure to stir it every once and while as it cools to stop the Shea butter from granulating.

Can I Heat Shea Butter?

Yes, you can heat Shea butter, but you have to know what you are doing. As discussed, Shea butter liquifies when it reaches body temperature without any loss of benefits. However, there are an abundance of videos on the internet showing you how to make your own whipped butter. Many of these show people liquifying the Shea butter to make it easier to whip. However, this is wrong! Subjecting Shea butter to extreme temperatures for a prolonged period of time will destroy the bioactive nutrients. It will still be useable, but the skin healing benefits will be gone.

Why Is My Shea Butter Hard?

Shea butter gets hard when it has been exposed to heat and then reforms. It could also be due to age. If your Shea butter is older than 18 months than it can turn hard and rancid.

My Shea Butter Stinks!

If you Shea butter has a bad smell it could be for multiple reasons. The most common reason is that the Shea butter was extracted using dirty water. The second reason is that the Shea butter has not been properly stored. The third reason is that the Shea nuts have been fermented before extraction. Lastly, your Shea butter could be extremely old and rancid and needs to be thrown away.

Where can I get good Shea Butter?

You can get quality Shea Butter products from Fra Fra's Naturals. We carry a wide variety of whipped Shea Butters and African Black Soaps. All of the Shea butter we carry is Grade A and certified Organic. Our Shea Butter products contain 97% raw Shea butter. While there are plenty of Shea butters on the market most manufactures are just adding just enough to be able to put Shea butter on the label. Don't be fooled by this.

BONUS:

10 DIY SKINCARE RECIPES

Skin care is an essential part of people's day. On average we use 10 different skin care products daily. While that doesn't seem bad the truth is that those products are loaded with chemicals. Our skin is the bodies largest organ. It acts as a barrier to the outside world keeping our internal organs safe. However, when it has been slathered with toxic chemicals it acts more like a sponge absorbing approximately 60% of what is put on it in as little as 26 seconds.

In recent years, there has been a bit of a green movement. People are becoming more concerned about what we are eating and how it is affecting us mentally and physically. It only makes sense that this "awakening" as extended to the beauty and skin care industry. Cosmetics companies tout these skin care products as safe for use and that may be true in small doses. But when used daily that toxicity builds up over time. It is a fact that there is little known about the long-term effects of most of these chemicals. However, we do know for certain that some chemicals are known dangers and can contribute to increased chances of birth defects, sperm damage, infertility, and some cancers.

There is a better way to take care of your skin, an all-natural way. You have just learned all about the wonderful properties and benefits of African black soap. Now let's put some of that knowledge to use and create some healthy—budget friendly—homemade body, hair skin care products that are free of chemical preservatives.

*Note: All these recipes require organic liquid or softened African black soap. To soften African black soap, grate a small piece of soap with a cheese grater. Add to a small pot and spray shavings with a small amount of water. Heat the pot on low. Stir and add water as needed until it has the consistency of Vaseline.

DIY NATURAL COFFEE EYE CREAM

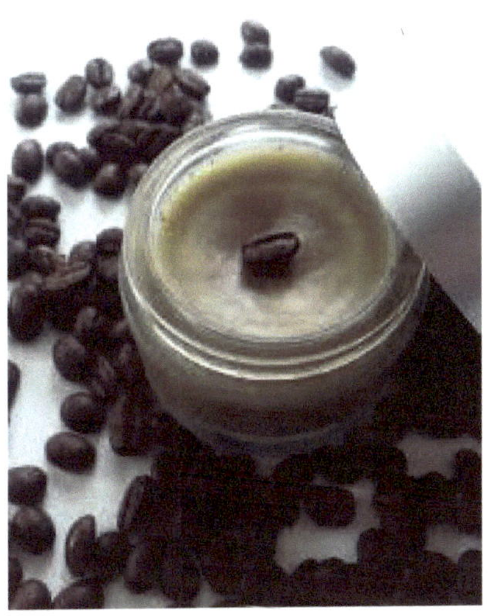

If you have a nightly skin care routine, then you know the importance of having a good eye cream. Eye creams moisturize, restore and hydrate the delicate under eye area overnight preventing dark circles. This recipe uses coffee and sweet almond oil because they are both great skin lightening agents. Coffee is naturally full of antioxidants which firms and tightens skin. It also increases blood circulation to give the skin a more rejuvenated and refreshed look. The Shea butter is added to reduce the inflammation that causes the appearance of puffy tired eyes.

What you will need:

- 1 tbsp coffee oil

- 2 tsp sweet almond oil

- 4 tsp of shea butter

- 4 tsp of cocoa butter

- 5 drops of vitamin E oil

- 5 drops of lavender essential oil (optional)

Directions:

Add softened shea butter, sweet almond oil and melted cocoa butter to a bowl. Mix in coffee oil along with vitamin E oil and lavender essential oil. Pour into a glass jar/container and let it set to harden. Gently pat around eyes before going to bed or in the morning under the eye makeup to brighten your eyes.

DIY PEPPERMINT FOOT CREAM

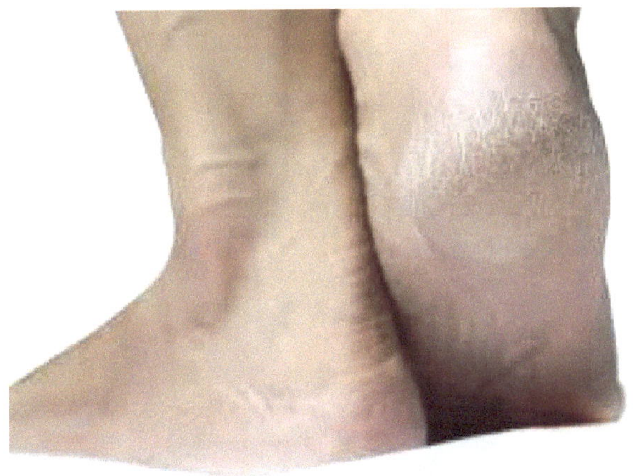

If your feet are in need of some pampering, then this is the recipe for you. This DIY whipped shea butter peppermint foot cream is easy to make, absorbs quickly and leaves your feet feeling refreshed.

What you will need:

- 1/3 cup shea butter

- 2 – 3 tbsp coconut oil

- 2 – 3 tbsp sweet almond oil

20-30 drops peppermint essential oil (varies by preference) Directions: Soften your shea butter by placing it in a bowl and placing that bowl in another bowl full of warm water or place the shea butter in the microwave on low. If you use the microwave, then keep it to short burst of 30 seconds each. Stir between each burst until shea butter is the right consistency. Stir in the remaining ingredients. Place mixture in the refrigerator or freezer to allow it to set. Once the mixture is firm (it will go from clear to opaque in color) whip it to a luxuriously fluffy texture with a hand blender. Transfer to an airtight container.

DIY SHEA BUTTER LIP BALM

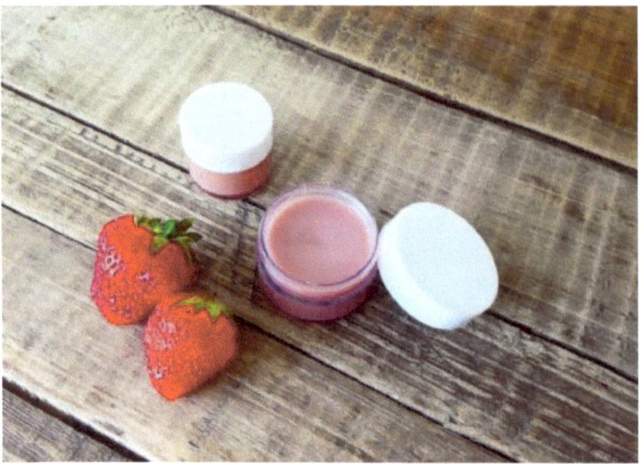

We often neglect our lips when we think of skincare, but our lips need care too. They get chapped, dried out and cracked. However, if you take care of your lips properly, they will be soft, healthy, and kissable.

What you will need:

- 2 tsp shea butter

- 2 tsp beeswax or soy wax pellets

- 2 tsp sweet almond oil

- 4 drops vitamin E oil

- 10-20 drops of essential oils (for flavor/optional)

- 1 tsp powdered herbs (Such as beetroot powder or alkanet root powder for color)

- Chapstick containers eye dropper

Directions:

Measure your oil and butter into a heatproof glass measuring cup and add your wax pellets. Set the glass measuring cup in a pan of gently boiling water to create a make-shift double boiler. The wax will melt last so be patient. Stir constantly. Be careful when removing the glass measuring cup as it will be very hot. Take a stainless-steel spoon and mix everything together. Pull the spoon out and wait a few minutes and see if the mixture on the spoon solidifies. Make sure it is not too hard for your lips or too soft to hold a shape.

Test this to see if it's hard or soft enough for your liking. Make your adjustments now (adding more oil if you want it softer, or more wax if you like it harder). If you opt to add the essential oils add it now along with the powdered herbs. Make sure there are no lumps. Stir and transfer the hot liquids into the directly into the lip balm containers.

DIY HYDRATING SHEA BUTTER FACE MASK

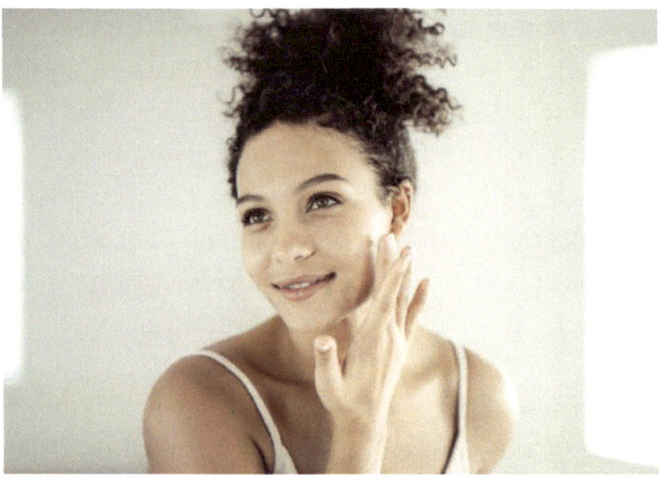

The skin is the largest organ of the human body. Anything that we put on our skin is absorbed into our bloodstream within 26 seconds. This is why it is so important to know what you are putting on your skin. It is my belief that what you put on your skin you should also be able to put in your mouth. This DIY face mask recipe is moisturizing, nourishing and full of shea buttery goodness.

What you will need:

- 2 tsp of shea butter
- 2 tsp sweet almond oil
- 1 tbsp aloe vera gel
- 2 -3 drops of essential oils (optional)
- Medium-sized bowl
-

Directions:

Place shea butter and sweet almond oil in a medium-sized bowl. Soften the mixture to make it easier to work with. Stir in the aloe vera gel and optional essential oils. The best oils for this mask are rose or lavender as

they help the skin absorb moisture deep into the lower dermis.
Before you apply this face mask you must first wash your face with a gentle cleanser. To optimize the effectiveness of this mask you should also do a mild scrub. Apply the mask to your face, neck and décolletage. Allow to sit for 10 -15 minutes then rinse.

GENTLE PAIN-RELIEVING SHEA BUTTER BALM

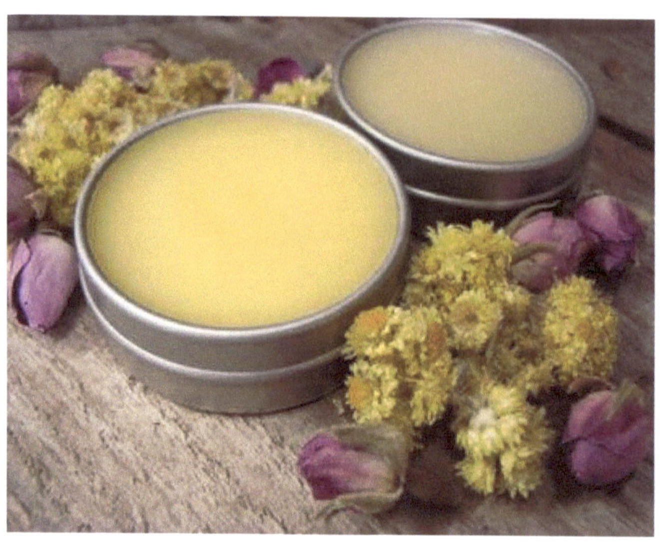

Everybody has little aches and pains. For some it just a small nuisance but for others it is constant discomfort. This DIY balm is made with Shea butter, Frankincense and Wintergreen essential oils.

Research shows that wintergreen oil has the ability to act like a natural analgesic (pain reducer), antiarthritic, antiseptic and astringent. North American tribes used Wintergreen to help cure fatigue, lung, sinuses, and respiratory ailments. Wintergreen oil has antioxidant properties and enhances the immune system as well as lower inflammation and reduce pain.

Traditionally, Priests, rabbis, and other medicine healers around the world used frankincense was used as incense in ancient rituals because of its promise to bring tremendous healing properties. Healers appreciated the oil for its antiseptic, anti-inflammatory and rejuvenating properties. Frankincense has a unique chemical makeup. It has an incredible high alpha-pinene content allowing it to work as an effective anti-inflammatory, anti-bacterial, anti-spasmodic, and analgesic good for alleviating pain associated with arthritis and other joint related issues.

Shea butter excellent at reducing inflammation. In African countries it has been used to provide relief for sore muscles for generations. This is because Shea butter has naturally occurring cinnamic acid in it. Cinnamic acid is what makes Shea butter so effective at diminishing inflammation when applied directly to sore joints and muscles.

What you will need:

- 3 tbsp beeswax pastilles

- 2 tbsp coconut oil

- 3 teaspoons sweet almond oil

- 8 drops spearmint essential oil

- 10 drops wintergreen essential oil

- 8 drops peppermint essential oil

- 8 drops frankincense essential oil

- Double Boiler (or a large pot & Mason jar)

Fill your double boiler or your pot with water up to just over half full. If you are using a pot place ingredient into a mason jar. Add the beeswax and bring water slowly to a boil. Stir wax, breaking it up. Be sure not to allow the wax to burn. Once the water has reached boiling turn the water back down to its lowest setting. Stir in the coconut oil and sweet almond oil. Once it is completely melted remove from heat and add the essential oils. Mix well and pour into your desired container. Leave the top off until it solidifies, and it completely cooled to room temperature. Place top on container and use as needed.

DIY MOISTURIZING SHAVING CREAM

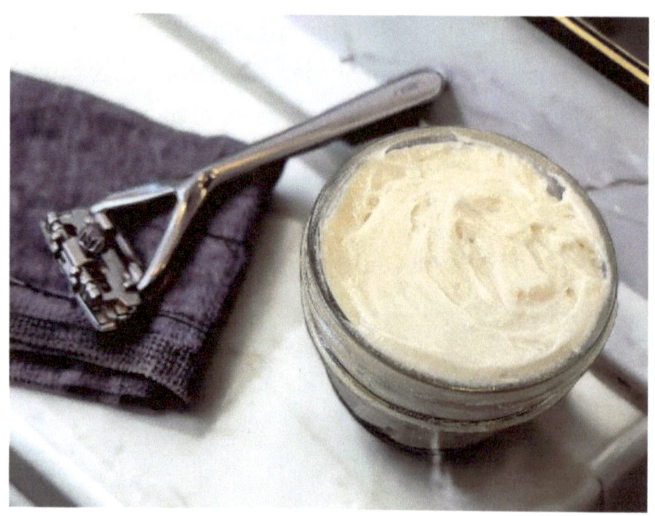

Shaving is a unisex endeavor. Shaving cream found on store shelves are full of chemicals and preservatives that can strip the skin and leave it irritated. A good alternative is a homemade shaving cream. It is cheaper to make, and you are completely in control of the ingredients. You might as well take care of your body. It is the only one you will ever get!

What you will need:

- 1/3 cup Shea butter

- 1/3 cup coconut oil

- 1/4 cup Extra-virgin olive oil

- 8 – 10 drops Peppermint essential oil

- 5 drops Lavender essential oil

Directions:

Place Shea butter and coconut oil in microwaveable bowl. Place it in microwave for about 30 seconds or until the mixture softens. Do not completely liquify the shea butter. Stir in the extra virgin olive oil and essential oils. Place in refrigerator to cool. This can take up to 2 hours. Once it solidifies take it out and let it sit for about 10 to 15 minutes. Take hand mixer or Wisk and beat until mixture is light and fluffy. Store in an airtight container in a cool dark place.

DIY CUTICLE CREAM

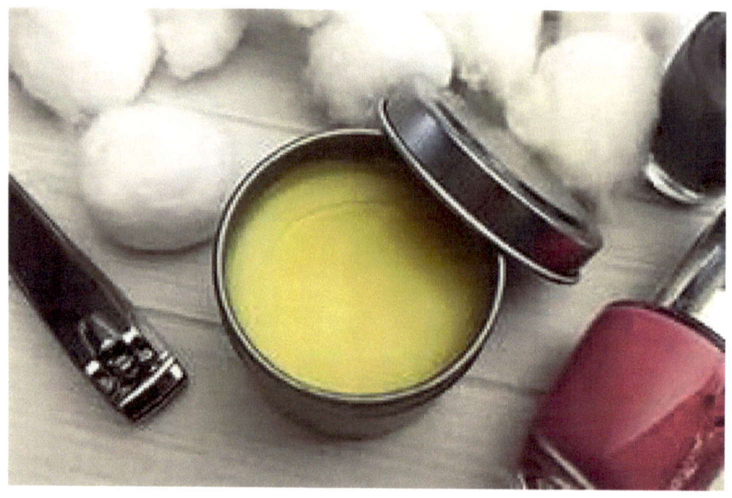

Cuticles are supposed to be soft. When exposed to harsh weather conditions or when you have just flat out neglected your nails your cuticles can pay the price. The problem with dry cuticles is that they crack, peel and bleed. It can also lead to a painful infection. To avoid dry cuticles, you should wear gloves when washing dishes and using cleaning products. You should also moisturize your cuticles daily. Below is an easy DIY cuticle cream to keep your nails and cuticles healthy and happy.

What you will need:

- 3 tbsp Shea butter

- 1 tbs beeswax pastilles

- 6 drops tea tree essential oil

- 6 drops lavender essential oil

Directions:

Melt beeswax in a double boiler or a mason jar sitting in a pan of simmering water. Add Shea butter and continue heating until Shea butter is softened and almost translucent. Remove from heat and stir in essential oils. Pour mixture into an airtight jar or container. Allow to cool completely before use.

DIY CURL CREAM

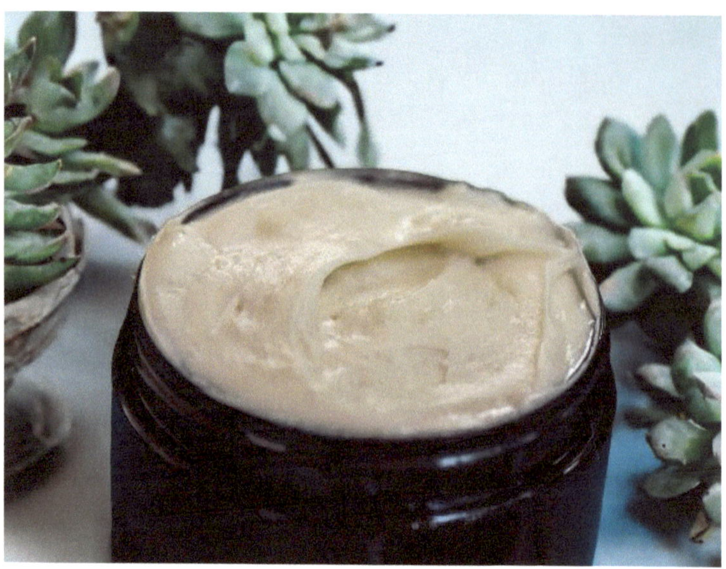

Curl cream is a moisturizing cream that is great for curly, thick, fine, or coarse hair, and it has moisturizing ingredients. This styling cream is not to thick or hard to apply. It absorbs quickly into the hair and allows you the flexibility of freshening up your hair throughout the day without dealing frizz or tangles.

What you will need:

- 2 tbsp shea butter

- ½ tbsp coconut oil

- ½ tbsp extra virgin olive oil

- ¾ tsp jojoba oil

- ¾ tsp sweet almond oil

- ½ tbsp aloe vera gel

- ⅛ tsp Vitamin E oil

- 6 drops rosemary essential oil

- 5 drops sandalwood essential oil 5 drops bergamot essential oil

Directions:

Combine shea butter and coconut oil in a glass measuring cup or half-pint mason jar. Soften in microwave for a few seconds. Mix in remaining ingredients. Transfer to desired jar or container with an airtight lid. Refrigerate until mixture is cooled and solidified. Remove from the refrigerator and store at room temperature.

CONCLUSION

In this guide, you have learned about all the amazing health benefits of raw shea butter. You have also learned about how to care for different skin types and how to use shea butter to address your skin care needs.

Shea butter is a natural emollient that can help to moisturize and protect the skin. It is also a good source of vitamins A and E, which are essential for skin health. Shea butter can help to reduce inflammation, soothe dry skin, and protect the skin from the sun's harmful rays.

Shea butter is safe for most people to use, but it is important to do a patch test before using it on a large area of skin. If you have any concerns, you should talk to your doctor or dermatologist.

Here are some tips for using shea butter in your daily skin care routine:

- Apply shea butter to your face and body after a shower or bath to lock in moisture.

- Use shea butter as a lip balm to keep your lips soft and smooth.

- Add a few drops of shea butter to your bathwater to create a relaxing and moisturizing soak.

- Make your own shea butter lotion by mixing shea butter with a carrier oil, such as coconut oil or almond oil.

Shea butter is a versatile and natural ingredient that can be used to improve the health and appearance of your skin. By following the tips in this guide, you can learn how to use shea butter to achieve your desired skin care goals.

Additionally, here are some of the ways that you can incorporate shea butter into your daily skin care routine:

- As a moisturizer: Shea butter is a great moisturizer for all skin types, including dry, sensitive, and acne-prone skin. It can help to hydrate the skin and prevent it from drying out.

- As a lip balm: Shea butter is a natural and effective lip balm that can help to keep your lips soft and smooth. It can also help to protect your lips from the elements.

- As a massage oil: Shea butter can be used as a massage oil to help relax muscles and relieve pain. It can also help to improve the appearance of scars and stretch marks.

- As a hair mask: Shea butter can be used as a hair mask to help moisturize and protect the hair. It can also help to reduce frizz and flyaways.

- As a makeup remover: Shea butter can be used as a makeup remover to gently remove makeup without stripping the skin's natural oils.

I hope this guide has helped you learn more about the wonders of shea butter. If you have any questions, please feel free to contact us.

We also carry a variety of organic raw unrefined shea butter, African black soap bars, and organic liquid African black soap on our website.

www.frafrasnaturals.com

We would love to hear from you!

FAQ ABOUT FRA FRA'S NATURALS

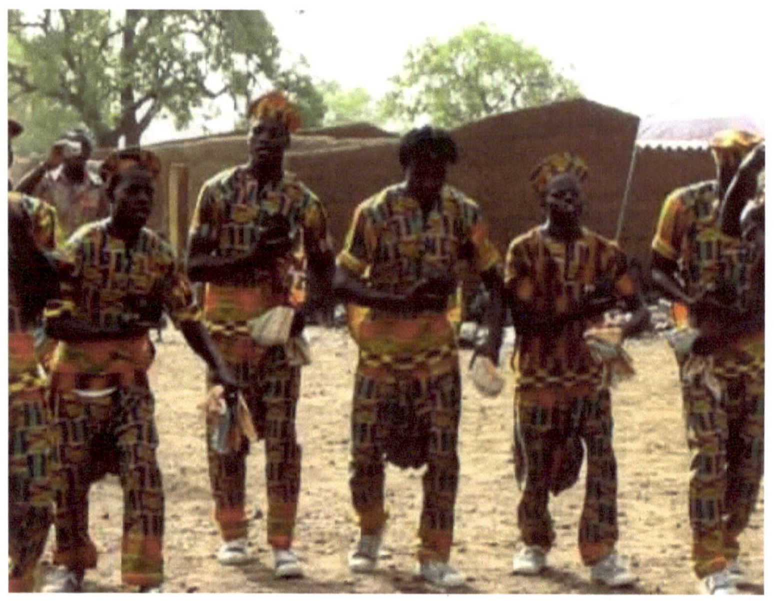

Q: Where does the name Fra Fra (pronounced fray fray) come from?

A: My husband's name is Frazier. When he was younger people called him Fra Fra. I recently found out there is a tribe in Northern Ghana, the primary source of Black Soap and Shea Butter, named the Fra Fra tribe. Once I began selling African black soap and shea butter, I knew that I would have to name our business Fra Fra's. I felt it was kismet.

Q: Who is the Fra Fra tribe?

A: The Fra Fra tribe is a subset of the Gur people living in northern Ghana. The name Fra Fra comes from the tribes traditional greeting "Ya Fara-Fara?", which means "How is your suffering (work)?" It is a sedentary agricultural tribe that grows all kinds of staples such as beans, maize, rice and yams. There are 300,000 Fra Fra speakers.

Q: I don't see the essential oil blend I need. Do you take request?

A: Yes! Please contact us if you would like for us to source an essential oil combination for you.

Q: Are you on social media?

A: Yes. Please follow us for exclusive sales and discounts:

@frafrasnaturals

Fra Fras Naturals Shea Butter and Black Soap

@frafrasnaturals

Frafrasnaturals